QUICK PSYCHOPHARMACOLOGY REFERENCE

MICHELE T. LARAIA, RN, MSN

Nursing Director of Research; Assistant Professor,
College of Medicine and College of Nursing,
Medical University of South Carolina,
Charleston, South Carolina

GAIL W. STUART, PhD, RN, CS

Chief, Division of Psychiatric Nursing; Professor,
College of Nursing, Associate Professor, College of Medicine,
Medical University of South Carolina,
Charleston, South Carolina

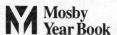

Mosby Year Book

St. Louis Baltimore Boston Chicago London Philadelphia Sydney Toronto

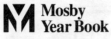

**Mosby
Year Book**

Dedicated to Publishing Excellence

Editor: Linda Duncan
Developmental Editor: Teri Merchant
Project Manager: Patricia Gayle May
Book and Cover Design: Gail Morey Hudson

Mosby–Year Book, Inc.
11830 Westline Industrial Drive, St. Louis, MO 63146

International Standard Book Number 0-8016-2729-X

CL/PC   9   8   7   6   5   4   3   2   1

CONTENTS

SECTION I **NURSING CARE GUIDELINES**

A. ROLE OF THE NURSE
1. Collection of pretreatment data
2. Coordination of treatment modalities
3. Patient education
4. Monitoring drug effects
5. Following psychopharmacological drug administration principles
6. Design of and participation in a drug maintenance program
7. Participation in concomitant nonpharmacological treatments
8. Participation in interdisciplinary clinical research drug trials

B. PRINCIPLES OF PATIENT ASSESSMENT
Psychiatric and medical history
Physical examination
Laboratory studies
Mental status evaluation
Diagnosis
Medication history
Family history
Treatment plan
Recording of dose, time, vital signs, observations
Result of drug administration

C. ESSENTIAL DOCUMENTATION

Drugs administered above daily recommended levels

Rationale for medication changes

Drugs used for other than the approved indications

Continued use of a drug that is causing clinically significant side effects

Polypharmacy rationale

Target symptoms and results of prn medications

Unusual concomitant prescribing

Critical adverse developments

Critical adjunctive services

D. MEDICATION ASSESSMENT TOOL

Psychiatric Medication

For each medication ever taken by the patient obtain the following information.

Name of drug

Why prescribed

Date started

Length of time taken

Highest daily dose

Who prescribed it?

Was it effective?

Side effects or adverse reactions

Was it taken as prescribed? (If not, explain).

Has anyone else in family been prescribed this drug?

If so, why was it prescribed and was it effective?

Prescription (Nonpsychiatric) Medications

For each medication taken by the patient in the past 6 months and for major medical illnesses if more than 6 months ago, obtain the following information.

Name of drug
Why prescribed
Date started
Highest daily dose
Who prescribed it?
Was it effective?
Side effects or adverse reactions
Was it taken as prescribed? (If not, explain.)

Over-the-Counter (Nonprescribed) Medications

For each medication taken by the patient in the past 6 months obtain the following information.

Name of drug
Why taken
Date started
Frequency of use
Was it effective?
Side effects or adverse reactions

Alcohol and Street Drugs

Name of substance
Date of first use
Frequency of use
Summarize effects
Adverse reactions

E. GUIDELINES FOR POLYPHARMACY

Identify specific target symptoms for each drug.

If possible, start with one drug and evaluate effectiveness and side effects before adding a second drug.

Be alert for adverse drug interactions.

Consider the effects of a second drug on the absorption and metabolism of the first drug.

Consider the possibility of additive side effects.

Change the dose of only one drug at a time and evaluate results.

Be aware of increased risk of medication errors.

Be aware of increased cost of treatment.

Be aware of decreased patient compliance in the aftercare setting when medication regimen is complex.

In follow-up treatment, eliminate as many drugs as possible, and establish the minimum effective dose of the drugs used.

Patient education programs regarding concomitant drug regimens must be particularly clear, organized, and effective.

Patient follow-up contacts should be more frequent.

F. INCREASED RISK FACTORS FOR PATIENT NONCOMPLIANCE

Failure to form a therapeutic alliance with the patient

Devaluation of pharmacotherapy by treatment staff

Inadequate patient and family education regarding treatment

Poorly controlled side effects

Insensitivity to patient complaints or wishes

Multiple daily dosing schedule

Polypharmacy

History of noncompliance

Social isolation

Expense of drugs

Failure to appreciate patient's role in drug treatment plan

Lack of continuity of care

Increased restrictions on patient's life-style

Unsupportive significant others

Remission of target symptoms

Increased suicidal ideation

Increased suspiciousness

Unrealistic expectations of drug effects

Failure to target residual symptoms for nonbiological therapies

Relapse or exacerbation of clinical syndrome

Failure to alleviate intrafamiliar and environmental stressors that precipitate symptoms

G. INTERACTIONS OF PSYCHOTROPIC DRUGS AND OTHER SUBSTANCES

Drug and category	Interacting drug or class	Possible consequences
Antipsychotic agents		
	Antacids, oral	Antacids may inhibit absorption of orally administered phenothiazines.
	CNS depressants Alcohol Barbiturates Antianxiety agents Antihistamines Narcotic analgesics	Additive CNS depression increases the risk of mental or physical impairment of performance.
	Anticholinergic agents; levodopa* (Bendopa, Larodopa, Levopa)	Additive atropine-like side effects may occur, antiparkinsonian effects of levodopa may be antagonized by antipsychotic agents.

Antianxiety agents

Benzodiazepines

CNS depressants
  Alcohol
  Barbiturates
  Antipsychotics
  Antihistamines

Additive CNS effects, especially sedation and decreased daytime performance, may occur.

Cimetidine

Cimetidine interferes with metabolism of long-acting benzodiazepines.

Antidepressant agents

Tricyclics

MAO inhibitors*

May cause hypertensive crisis if tricyclic is added to MAO inhibitors.

Alcohol, other central nervous system depressants

Acute use causes additive CNS depression; *chronic use* may increase tricyclic metabolism.

Antihypertensives*
  Guanethidine (Ismelin)
  Methyldopa (Aldomet)
  Clonidine (Catapres)

Antagonism of antihypertensive effects may occur with loss of control of blood pressure.

Antipsychotics
Anticholinergics

Additive atropine-like effects may occur.

Continued.

7

G. INTERACTIONS OF PSYCHOTROPIC DRUGS AND OTHER SUBSTANCES—cont'd

Drug and category	Interacting drug or class	Possible consequences
	Antiarrhythmics Quinidine Procainamide	Additive antiarrhythmic effects, prolongation of QRS complex may occur.
Mood stabilizer Lithium	Diuretics* Hydrochlorothiazide	Diuretic-induced sodium depletion can increase lithium levels; may cause toxicity.
	Nonsteroidal antiinflammatory agents* Ibuprofen Indomethacin Phenylbutazone	Lithium blood levels are increased; may cause toxicity.

*Potentially clinically significant.

H. INCREASED RISK FACTORS FOR DEVELOPMENT OF DRUG INTERACTIONS

Polypharmacy
High doses
Geriatric patients
Debilitated/dehydrated patients
Concurrent illness
Compromised organ system function
Inadequate patient education
History of noncompliance
Failure to include patient in treatment planning

ANTIANXIETY AND SEDATIVE-HYPNOTIC DRUGS

COMMON INDICATIONS
Anxiety
Sedation/sleep
Neuroleptic-induced akathisia
Muscle spasms
Seizure disorders
Toxic psychoses caused by hallucinogenic drugs
Alcohol withdrawal syndromes

BENZODIAZEPINES

Generic name	Trade name	Dose (mg/day)
Antianxiety drugs		
Alprazolam	Xanax	0.5-4
Chlordiazepoxide	Librium	20-100
Chlorazepate	Tranxene	7.5-60
Diazepam	Valium	10-40
Halazepam	Paxipam	80-160
Lorazepam	Ativan	2-6
Oxazepam	Serax	15-90
Prazepam	Centrax	10-60
Sedative-hypnotic drugs		
Flurazepam	Dalmane	15-60
Temazepam	Restoril	15-30
Triazolam	Halcion	0.25-0.5

NONBENZODIAZEPINE

Generic name	Trade name	Dose (mg/day)
Buspirone	Buspar	10-40

BENZODIAZEPINE SIDE EFFECTS AND NURSING CONSIDERATIONS

Side effects	Nursing considerations
Acute/common	
Drowsiness, sedation	Activity helps; caution when using machinery
Ataxia, dizziness	Caution with activity, prevent falls
Feelings of detachment	Discourage social isolation
Increased irritability or hostility	Observe carefully, offer support, be alert for disinhibition of control over socially unacceptable impulses
Anterograde amnesia	Inability to recall events that occur while the drug is active; desirable in preoperative use
Long-term/common	
Minor tolerance to some effects	Short-term use if possible; discontinue, using a slow taper; not recommended for use with people with history of drug or alcohol abuse
Dependency	
Rebound insomnia/anxiety	

Rare (causal relationship uncertain)

Increased appetite and weight gain	Weight control measures
Cutaneous reactions	Usually not clinically significant
Nausea	Dose with meals, decrease dose
Headache	Usually responds to mild analgesic
Confusion	Decrease dose
Gross psychomotor impairment	Dose-related, decrease dose
Depression	Decrease dose; may require antidepressant treatment
Paradoxical rage reaction	Discontinue drug

NURSE NOTE

The benzodiazepines generally do not live up to their reputation of being strongly addictive if their discontinuation is accomplished by gradual tapering, if they have been used for appropriate purposes, and if their use has not been complicated by the use of other substances, such as chronic use of barbiturates or alcohol. Watch particularly for:

1. Sedation
2. Ataxia
3. Irritability
4. Memory problems

Well absorbed when given orally on an empty stomach.

Antacids seriously interfere with absorption.

IM use varies by drug and site: diazepam and lorazepam are reliably absorbed if given in the deltoid muscle; chlordiazepoxide is not absorbed IM and is never given by this route.

IV use is rare in psychiatric practice; IV diazepam or lorazepam is used if anticholinergics fail to treat neuroleptic-induced laryngeal dystonias, and in some agitated or delirious states for emergency sedation; must be given slowly over the space of a minute or two rather than rapid push because of the risk of respiratory depression at peak levels.

Metabolized in the liver; thus routine doses could lead to toxicity in patients with liver dysfunction.

Use in pregnancy: there are no prospective studies to demonstrate that benzodiazepines are safe; there are anecdotal reports, though unsubstantiated, that first-trimester use causes oral cleft abnormalities.

Nonbenzodiazepines, with the exception of buspirone, are rarely used in psychiatry today because of their many disadvantages:

they are more addictive, tolerance develops, they have dangerous withdrawal symptoms, they are dangerous in overdose, and they have a variety of dangerous drug interactions. Barbiturates are examples of these drugs.

BENZODIAZEPINE WITHDRAWAL SYNDROME

Usually worsens several days after taper begins, and increases over several weeks, then subsides. Minimize by slowing taper.

Mild symptoms	Severe symptoms
Tremulousness	Diarrhea
Insomnia	Hypotension
Dizziness	Hyperthermia
Headaches	Neuromuscular irritability
Tinnitus	Psychosis
Anorexia	Seizures
Vertigo	
Blurred vision	
Agitation	
Anxiety	

CONTRAINDICATIONS

History of chemical dependency/substance abuse
Open-ended treatment with no assessment for further need
Failure to use nonpharmacological therapies when indicated

ADJUNCTIVE SERVICES

Benzodiazepine drug screens

SECTION III   ANTIDEPRESSANT DRUGS: CYCLIC ANTIDEPRESSANTS AND MONOAMINE OXIDASE INHIBITORS (MAOIs)

COMMON INDICATIONS
Depression
Bipolar depression
Panic disorder
Bulimia
Neuropathic pain
Enuresis

POSSIBLY EFFECTIVE
Attention-deficit-hyperactivity disorder
Organic affective disorders
Obsessive-compulsive disorder
Posttraumatic stress disorder
Conduct disorder in children
School phobia and separation disorder

ANTIDEPRESSANT DRUGS

Generic name	Trade name	Dose (mg/day)
Tricyclic drugs		
Amitriptyline	Elavil, Endep	50-300
Amoxapine	Asendin	50-600
Doxepin	Adapin, Sinequan	50-300
Imipramine	SK-Pramine, Tofranil	50-300
Trimipramine	Surmontil	50-300
Desipramine	Norpramin, Pertofrane	50-300
Nortriptyline	Aventyl, Pamelor	50-150
Protriptyline	Vivactil	15-60
Nontricyclic drugs		
Maprotiline	Ludiomil	50-225*
Fluoxetine	Prozac	20-80
Trazodone	Desyrel	50-600
Buproprion	Wellbutrin	50-600*
Monoamine oxidase inhibitors		
Isocarboxazid	Marplan	30-70
Phenelzine	Nardil	45-90
Tranylcypromine	Parnate	20-60

*Antidepressants with a ceiling dose because of dose-related seizures.

SIDE EFFECTS AND NURSING CONSIDERATIONS

Side effects	Nursing considerations
Orthostatic hypotension (dizziness, lightheadedness)	Assess risk of falls; caution patient to rise slowly; assess vital signs standing and sitting
Anticholinergic effects (dry mouth, blurred vision, constipation, excessive sweating, urinary hesitancy/retension, tacchycardia, agitation, delirium, exacerbation of glaucoma)	Adequate hydration, caution when using machinery, fiber-rich diet, assess mentation, assess for cardiac toxicity if history is positive for conduction system disease
Neurological effects (sedation, psychomotor slowing, poor concentration, fatigue, tremors, ataxia)	Advise caution when using machinary; dose HS unless insomnia occurs; lower dose and titrate up more slowly
Miscellaneous (decreased libido and sexual performance)	Separate last dose and sexual intercourse by as many hours as possible; reduce dose

DIETARY RESTRICTIONS 1 DAY BEFORE, DURING, AND 2 WEEKS AFTER TAKING MAOIs*

Food and Beverages to Avoid

Cheese, especially aged or matured
Fermented or aged protein
Pickled or smoked fish
Beer, red wine, sherry, liqueurs, cognac
Yeast or protein extacts
Fava or broad bean pods
Beef or chicken liver
Spoiled or overripe fruit
Banana peel
Yogurt

Food and Beverages to be Consumed in Moderation

Chocolate
Yogurt and sour cream
Clear spirits and white wine
Avocado
New Zealand spinach
Soy sauce
Caffeine drinks

---

*Modified from Zisook, S.: Psychosomatics 26(3):240-251, March 1985, and Moreines, R., and Gold, M.S.: In Gold, M.S., Lydiard, R.B., and Carman, J.S., editors: Advances in psychopharmacology: predicting and improving treatment response, Boca Raton, Fla., 1984, CRC Press.

Safe Food and Beverages

Fresh cottage cheese
Cream cheese
Fresh fruits
Bread products raised with yeast (bread)

Medications to Avoid

Cold medications
Nasal and sinus decongestants
Allergy and hay fever remedies
Narcotics, especially meperidine
Inhalants for asthma
Local anesthetics with epinephrine
Weight-reducing pills, pep pills, stimulants
Other medications without first checking with a physician

Illicit Drugs to Avoid

Cocaine
Amphetamine

Safe Medications

Aspirin, acetaminophen
Pure steroid asthma inhalants
Codeine
Plain quaifenesin or terpin hydrate with codeine
Local anesthetics without epinephrine
All laxatives
All antibiotics
Antihistamines

Medications That May Need Dose Decreased

Insulin and oral hypoglycemics
Oral anticoagulants
Thiazide diuretics
Anticholinergic agents
Muscle relaxants

SIGNS AND TREATMENT OF HYPERTENSIVE CRISIS IN MAOI THERAPY

Warning Signs

Increased blood pressure, palpitations, frequent headaches

Symptoms of Hypertensive Crisis

Sudden elevation of blood pressure
Explosive headache, occipital that may radiate frontally
Head and face are flushed and feel "full"
Palpitations, chest pain
Sweating, fever
Nausea, vomiting
Dilated pupils
Photophobia
Intracranial bleeding

Treatment

Hold next MAOI dose
Do not let patient lie down (elevates blood pressure in head)
IM chlorpromazine 100 mg, repeat if necessary (*mechanism of action:* blocks norepinephine)
IV phentolamine, administered slowly in doses of 5 mg (*mechanism*

of action: binds with norepinephrine receptor sites, blocking norepinephrine)

Fever: Manage by external cooling techniques

NURSE NOTE

Tricyclic antidepressants have a 3- to 4-week delay before therapeutic response.

They have no known long-term adverse effects.

Tolerance to therapeutic effects does not develop.

Persistent side effects can often be minimized by a small decrease in
dose.

These drugs do not cause physical addiction or psychological depen-
dence.

They do not cause euphoria; thus they have no abuse potential.

They can be conveniently dosed once a day.

Cyclic medications are usually the first choice of treatment because
of their established effectiveness, relative safety, and ease of administration.

MAOIs are generally used for cyclic nonresponders or cyclic-intol-
erant patients because of concern regarding the need for dietary
restrictions.

Cyclic antidepressants and buproprion lower the seizure threshold;
MAOIs do not.

A careful evaluation of suicide risk must be taken of all depressed
patients because all these drugs have a narrow therapeutic index
and can be lethal in overdose (trazodone and fluoxetine are excep-
tions).

Use during pregnancy; cyclic antidepressants: although there is no
compelling evidence that cyclic antidepressants cause congenital

malformations, their use during pregnancy should be avoided unless the pregnant woman is at risk for life-threatening depression.

Use during pregnancy; MAOIs: there is little information regarding safety; thus they are best avoided.

All these drugs are in oral form; amitriptyline and imipramine are also in IM form.

CONTRAINDICATIONS

Allergy to these drugs

Cyclics: cardiac conduction system disease

MAOIs: inability to follow dietary restriction

ADJUNCTIVE SERVICES

Dexamethasone suppression test (DST) >5 ng/ml is positive

Tricyclic blood levels	(ng/ml)
Imipramine	>225
Desipramine	>125
Amitriptyline	>120 (?)*
Nortriptyline	>50-150
Doxepin	>100-250 (?)*

* Technology uncertain.

SECTION IV MOOD-STABILIZING DRUGS

COMMON INDICATIONS
Acute mania
Bipolar prophylaxis

PROBABLY EFFECTIVE
Unipolar prophylaxis

POSSIBLY EFFECTIVE
Bulimia
Alcohol abuse
Aggressive behaviors
Schizoaffective disorder

LITHIUM

Generic name	Trade name	Available forms
Lithium carbonate	Eskalith	150, 300 mg
	PFI-Lith	
	Lithotabs	
	Lithane	
	Lithonate	
Lithium carbonate, sustained-release	Lithobid	300 mg
	Eskalith C-R	450 mg
Lithium citrate, concentrate	Ciba-Lith	5 ml/300 mg
	Lithonate-S	

PRELITHIUM WORK-UP

Renal

Urinalysis, BUN, creatinine, electrolytes, 24-hour creatinine clearance; history of renal disease in self or family; diabetes mellitus, hypertension, diuretic use, analgesic abuse

Thyroid

TSH (thyroid-stimulating hormone), T_4 (thyroxine), T_3 RU (resin uptake), T_4 I (free thyroxine index); history of thyroid disease in self or family

Other

Complete physical, history; ECG, fasting blood sugar, CBC

STABILIZING LITHIUM LEVELS

Common Causes for an Increase in Lithium Levels

Decreased sodium intake
Diuretic therapy
Decreased renal functioning
Fluid and electrolyte loss: sweating, diarrhea, dehydration
Medical illness
Overdose

Ways to Maintain a Stable Lithium Level

Stable dosing schedule by dividing doses or use of sustained-release
    capsules
Adequate dietary sodium and fluid intake (2 to 3 quarts/day)
Replace fluid and electrolytes during exercise or GI illness
Monitor signs and symptoms of lithium side effects and toxicity
If patient forgets a dose, he may take it if he missed dosing time by
    2 hours; if longer than 2 hours, skip that dose and take the next
    dose; never double up on doses

LITHIUM SIDE EFFECTS

Acute/Common/Usually Harmless

CNS: Fine hand tremor (50% of patients), fatigue, headache, mental
    dullness, lethargy
Renal: Polyuria (60% of patients), polydipsia, edema
Gastrointestinal: Gastric irritation, anorexia, abdominal cramps,
    mild nausea, vomiting, diarrhea (dose with food or milk; further
    divide dose)
Dermatologic: Acne, pruritic maculopapular rash

Cardiac: ECG changes, usually not clinically significant, may be persistent

Body image: Weight gain (60% of patients); can be persistent

Long-Term/Adverse/Usually Not Dose Related (Patient Usually Can Remain on Lithium)

Endocrine

Thyroid dysfunction—hypothyroidism (5% of patients); replacement hormone may be necessary

Mild diabetes mellitus—may need diet control or insulin therapy

Renal

Nephrogenic diabetes insipidus—decreasing dose can help; patient must drink plently of fluids; thiazide diuretics paradoxically reduce polyuria and may be helpful

Microscopic structural kidney changes: (10%-20% of patients on lithium for 1 year); usually does not cause significant clinical morbidity

Lithium Toxicity/Usually Dose Related

Prodrome of intoxication (lithium level $\geq$2.0 mEq/l)

Anorexia, nausea, vomiting, diarrhea, coarse hand tremor, muscle fasciculations, twitching, lethargy, dysarthria, hyperactive deep tendon reflexes, ataxia, tinnitus, vertigo, weakness, drowsiness

Lithium intoxication (lithium level $\geq$2.5 mEq/l)

Fever, decreased urine output, decreased BP, irregular pulse, EKG changes, impaired consciousness, seizures, coma, death

MANAGEMENT OF SERIOUS LITHIUM TOXICITY

1. Rapid assessment of clinical signs and symptoms of lithium toxicity; if possible, obtain rapid history of incident, especially

dosing, from patient; explain procedures to patient and offer support throughout

2. Hold all lithium doses
3. Check blood pressure, pulse, rectal temperature, respirations, level of consciousness. Be prepared to: initiate stabilization procedures, protect airway, provide supplemental oxygen
4. Obtain lithium blood level immediately; obtain electrolytes, BUN, creatinine, urinalysis, CBC when possible
5. Electrocardiogram; monitor cardiac status
6. Limit lithium absorption; if acute overdose, provide an emetic; nasogastric suctioning may help because lithium levels in gastric fluid may remain high for days
7. Vigorously hydrate: 5 to 6 L/day; keep electrolytes balanced; IV line and indwelling urinary catheter
8. Patient will be bedridden: range of motion, frequent turning, pulmonary toilet
9. In moderately severe cases:
    a. Implement osmotic diuresis with urea, 20 g IV two to five times per day, or mannitol, 50 to 100 g IV per day
    b. Increase lithium clearance with aminophylline, 0.5 g up to every 6 hours, and alkalinize the urine with IV sodium lactate
    c. Ensure adequate intake of NaCl to promote excretion of lithium
    d. Implement peritoneal or hemodialysis in the most severe cases. These are characterized by serum levels between 2.0 and 4.0 mEq/L with severe clinical signs and symptoms (particularly decreasing urinary output and deepening CNS depression).
10. When appropriate: interview patient; ascertain reasons for lithium toxicity; increase health teaching efforts; mobilize postdis-

charge support system; arrange for more frequent clinical visits and blood levels; assess for depression and/or suicidal intent; consider concomitant antidepressant drug treatment and supportive nonpharmacologic therapy

NURSE NOTE

Lithium is excreted almost entirely by the kidneys; thus kidney function must be adequate.

Lithium comes in oral tablets, capsules, and liquid.

Lithium toxicity is a life-threatening emergency.

Blood levels must be monitored frequently.

Lithium can be combined with other antidepressant and antipsychotic drugs.

Patients need careful education about maintenance of lithium levels.

Hold lithium dose if toxicity is suspected.

Use in pregnancy: associated with cardiac anomalies when used during the first trimester; use later in pregnancy may complicate lithium levels for the mother because of changes in maternal blood volume; thus best to avoid during pregnancy.

MAINTENANCE LITHIUM CONSIDERATIONS

Every 3 months: Lithium level (for the first 6 months)

Every 6 months: reassess renal status, lithium level, TSH

Every 12 months: reassess thyroid function, ECG

Assess more often if patient is symptomatic or if toxicity is suspected.

ADJUNCTIVE SERVICES

Lithium Levels

Draw level 12 hours after last dose, usually in AM before first dose of the day; 1.0-1.2 mEq/L for acute mania.

Draw every 5 days to adjust dose initially.
Draw less frequently as levels stabilize.

ANTICONVULSANT DRUGS USED AS MOOD STABILIZERS

Generic name	Trade name	Dosage (mg/day)
Carbamazepine	Tegretol	200-1600
Valproic acid	Valproate	800-1800
Clonazepam	Klonopin	2-16

SIDE EFFECTS OF CARBAMAZEPINE

Common, Dose-Related

Dizziness
Ataxia
Clumsiness
Sedation
Dysarthria
Diplopia
Nausea and GI upset
Reversible mild leukopenia

Less Common, Dose-Related

Tremor
Memory disturbance
Confusional states
Cardiac conduction disturbances

Idiosyncratic Toxicities (Rare)

Rash (including cases of exfoliation)
Lenticular opacities
Hepatitis
Blood dyscrasias
    Aplastic anemia
    Leukopenia
    Thrombocytopenia

NURSE NOTE FOR CARBAMAZEPINE

Carbamazepine comes in oral form only.

Serum levels for bipolar disorder: 8-12 µg/ml.

Increase doses slowly, and use the minimum effective level to minimize side effects.

Recommendations for hematological monitoring

    CBC before treatment, follow patients with baseline abnormalities closely.

    Check blood counts every 2 weeks during the first 2 months of treatment.

    Monitor for symptoms of bone marrow suppression.

    Check every 3 months after that if no abnormalities appear.

    Stop drug if WBC drops below 3000/mm^3 or neutrophil count goes below 1500/mm^3.

Overdose: There are no reported fatalities from this drug alone.

Use in pregnancy: Effects are unknown; thus the drug should be avoided.

SIDE EFFECTS AND NURSING CONSIDERATIONS FOR VALPROIC ACID

Side effects	Nursing considerations
Nausea	Administer with food
Hepatotoxicity (transient SGOT and SGPT elevations; severe hepatitis (rare): malaise anorexia, or jaundice)	Discontinue drug immediately
Neurotoxicity (sedation, hand tremor, ataxia)	
Hematologic toxicity (thrombocytopenia or platelet dysfunction)	Check platelet count and bleeding time before any surgery
Pancreatitis (rare)	

NURSE NOTE FOR VALPROIC ACID

Used in bipolar disorder both as a single agent or in combination with lithium.

Optimal blood levels are thought to be in the range of 40-150 μg/ml in seizure disorders; they are unknown in bipolar disorder.

Contraindicated in patients with known liver disease;

Use in pregnancy: little human data exists, but this drug is teratogenic in animals; thus it is contraindicated in pregnancy;

Initiate slowly to minimize side effects.

NURSE NOTE FOR CLONAZEPAM

This is a benzodiazepine used to treat anxiety. Case reports suggest efficacy in acute mania.

Suggested use is for lithium- or carbamazepine-resistant manic patients.

May be effective in blocking panic attacks (preliminary reports; dose at 1.5 to 5 mg/day).

Side effects include sedation, development of tolerance, paradoxical excitement.

SECTION V ANTIPSYCHOTIC DRUGS

COMMON INDICATIONS
Psychotic symptoms of schizophrenia, acute mania, depression, and
   toxic and organic conditions
Gilles de la Tourette disorder
Treatment-resistant bipolar disorder
Huntington's disease and other movement disorders

POSSIBLY EFFECTIVE
Paranoid disorders
Childhood psychoses

NONPSYCHIATRIC USES
Nausea and vomiting
Intractable hiccups
Preanesthesia

ANTIPSYCHOTIC DRUGS

Generic name	Trade name	Dose (mg/day)
Chlorpromazine	Thorazine	300-1400
Thioridazine	Mellaril	300-800*
Mesoridazine	Serentil	100-500
Perphenazine	Trilafon	8-64
Trifluoperazine	Stelazine	10-80
Fluphenazine	Prolixin	5-40
Thiothixene	Navane	10-60
Haloperidol	Haldol	5-100
Loxapine	Loxitane	50-250
Molindone	Moban	25-250
Clozapine	Clozaril	300-600

*Upper limit to avoid retinopathy

ANTIPSYCHOTIC DRUG SIDE EFFECTS AND NURSING CONSIDERATIONS

Side effects and adverse reactions	Treatment and nursing considerations
Acute, common side effects	
Neurological	General EPS treatment principles:
	1. Tolerance usually develops by the third month.
	2. Decrease dose of antipsychotic drug if possible.
	3. Add an anticholinergic drug for 3 months, then taper.
	4. Provide patient education and supportive care.
Extrapyramidal symptoms (EPS)	
1. Acute dystonic reactions occur suddenly and are frightening to the patient. Spasms of major muscle groups of the neck, back, and eyes; catatonia; and respiratory compromise occur.	Administer an anticholinergic drug; have respiratory support equipment available.

36

2. Akathisia is characterized by pacing, inner restlessness and leg aches, which are relieved by movement.

   Rule out anxiety or agitation (difficult but important distinction)

3. Parkinson's syndrome is characterized by:

   a. Akinesia— absence or slowness of motion; patient turning like one solid block of wood; gait inclined forward with small, rapid steps; masklike facies

   b. Cogwheel rigidity and muscle stiffness on physical exam

   c. Bilateral fine tremor, anywhere in body; "pill-rolling" motion of the fingers

   Tolerance does not develop in all patients; the dopamine agonist, amantadine, is sometimes effective (patient must have good renal function to avoid amantadine toxicity); use principle 3 (above) early and vigorously.

Continued.

37

ANTIPSYCHOTIC DRUG SIDE EFFECTS AND NURSING CONSIDERATIONS—cont'd

Side effects and adverse reactions	Treatment and nursing considerations
Behavioral Sleepiness, grogginess, fatigue	Tolerance occurs within days to several weeks; rule out overmedication; dose once daily at hs; change to an antipsychotic drug with a lower sedation profile.
Autonomic Blurred vision, constipation, tachycardia, urinary retention, decreased gastric secretion, decreased sweating and salivation (dry mouth), heat stroke, nasal congestion, decreased pulmonary secretion; "atropine psychosis" in geriatric patients: hyperactivity, agitation, confusion, flushed skin, dilated pupils that are slow to react, bowel hypomotility, dysarthria	Tolerance develops in days to weeks; treat symptomatically; frequently moisten dry mouth, use sugarless candy and gum; bulk diets, stool softeners, fluids, and exercise for constipation; avoid operating machinery if vision is blurred; cholinergic agonist (bethanechol) for urinary retention; IM physostigmine for severe atropine psychosis; avoid polypharmacy if possible; avoid getting overheated.

Cardiac (autonomic)
Dizziness, tachycardia, drop in diastolic BP by >40 mm Hg with a change of position from lying to sitting or sitting to standing

Tolerance develops in several weeks; lower dose; change to an antipsychotic with lower hypotension profile, monitor BP; increase fluid intake to expand vascular volume; have patient rise slowly and dangle feet while sitting; have patient wear support hose.

Long-term, common side effects
Neurological
Extrapyramidal symptom (EPS)
Tardive dyskinesia; tongue protrusion, lip smacking, puckering, sucking, chewing, blinking, lateral jaw movements, grimacing; choreoid movements of the limbs and trunk, shoulder shrugging, pelvic thrusting, wrist and ankle flexion or rotation, foot tapping, toe movements

These are stereotyped, involuntary movements that may be mild or become severely crippling; employ primary preventive measures; patients with severe tardive dyskinesia can become distressed; may need soft foods, and soft shoes for feet movements. There is no treatment for tardive dyskinesia, though several drugs are in the experimental stages; may be irreversible, especially if not discovered early and if antipsychotic drugs cannot be stopped.
Continued.

ANTIPSYCHOTIC DRUG SIDE EFFECTS AND NURSING CONSIDERATIONS—cont'd

Side effects and adverse reactions	Treatment and nursing considerations
Short- or long-term, rare, life-threatening side effects *Neuroleptic malignant syndrome* High fever, tachycardia, muscle rigidity, stupor, tremor, incontinence, leukocytosis, elevated serum CPK, hyperkalemia, renal failure, increased pulse, respirations, and sweating	This is an *extreme emergency*—early recognition is critical; avoid marked dehydration in all patients; discontinue all drugs immediately; give supportive symptomatic care; nutrition, hydration, renal dialysis for renal failure, ventilation for acute respiratory failure, reduction of fever. *Speculative:* dantrolene, bromocriptine. Antipsychotic drugs can be cautiously reintroduced.

DRUGS TO TREAT ANTIPSYCHOTIC EXTRAPYRAMIDAL SIDE EFFECTS

Generic name	Trade name	Dose (mg/day)
Anticholinergic		
Benztropine	Cogentin	1-6
Trihexyphenidyl	Artane	1-10
Biperiden	Akineton	2-6
Procyclidine	Kemadrin	6-20
Dopaminergic		
Amantadine	Symmetrel	100-300
Gabaminergic		
Diazepam	Valium	5-40
Lorazepam	Ativan	2-10
Antihistamines		
Diphenhydramine	Benadryl	25-100
Orphenadrine	Norflex	50-300

NURSE NOTES

Liquid preparations are absorbed more rapidly and reliably than tablets; parenterally administered antipsychotics are rapidly and reliably absorbed.

All of the antipsychotic drugs are equivalent in efficacy (maximal therapeutic effect), but differ in potency (amount of drug needed to achieve that effect); thus they differ in side effect profile.

After initial divided doses, can dose once a day;

Food or antacids may decrease absorption;

There are two long-lasting IM preparations: fluphenazine allows administration every 2 weeks, and haloperidol allows dosing intervals of 4 weeks.

Relatively safe in overdose situations when used alone.

Use in pregnancy: not recommended because of lack of safety data unless lack of treatment of the mother presents a greater risk to the fetus than possible drug effects.

Check for tardive dyskinesia with the abnormal involuntary movement scale (AIMS) once a month in long-term treatment.

REFERENCES

Bouricius JK: Psychoactive drugs and their effects on mentally ill persons, National Alliance for the Mentally Ill, Publications No. 3, Second Series, 1989, Arlington, Virginia.

Hyman SE and Arana GW: Handbook of psychiatric drug therpay, Boston, 1987, Little Brown and Co.

Laraia MT: Psychopharmacology. In Stuart GW and Sundeen SJ: Principles and practice of psychiatric nursing, ed 4, St. Louis, 1991, Mosby–Year Book, Inc.

Stuart GW and Sundeen SJ: Pocket guide to psychiatric nursing, St. Louis, 1991, Mosby–Year Book, Inc.

Towery OB and Brands AB: Psychotropic drugs: approaches to psychopharmacologic drug use, US Department of Health and Human Services, NIH, Rockville, Md, 1980.